Unhappy Patients

A Look at Dental Patients' Complaints About Their Dental Care

Curtis F. Smith, DDS, FACD, FICD

2018

First Edition
Unhappy Patients
Copyright 2018 © Curtis F. Smith
All rights reserved.

ISBN 978-0-692-10388-3

Prepress specialist: Kathleen R. Weisel
(weiselcreative.com)

Dedication

There is a self-description of dentistry within the profession that is revealing. "We invade an emotionally charged personal space, perform mostly uncomfortable procedures, and then charge you for it."

To all those patients who put up with it and don't complain, this book is dedicated.

Contents

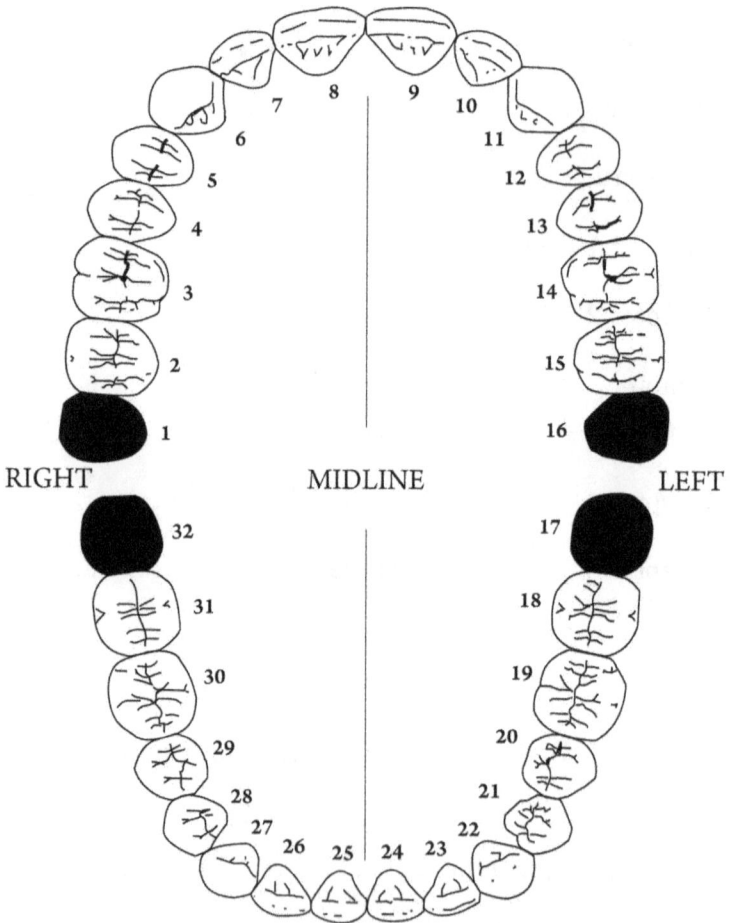

RIGHT   MIDLINE   LEFT

Image: Burak Duman, fotolia.us

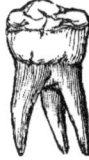

Introduction

This is how I came to be reading, analyzing and making recommendations on three or four or five patient complaints a week:

The company I worked for is the largest dental insurer in the state. They cover more than two million insured persons and their dependents. Because the company has several national accounts, it covers patients in more than 40 states. The network of member dental offices in the states includes more the 80% of the licensed dentists.

Employers purchasing dental coverage for their employees want to be sure that the money is well spent and that the dental care delivered is of high quality. For that reason, the company has developed a Quality Management (QM) process for evaluating complaints that come to them involving member dentists.

A dentist receives the complaint, makes a summary of the facts and produces a recommendation. The QM Committee then discusses the case and makes a decision. Complaints often ask for apologies from the dentist involved, monetary damages, compensation for pain and suffering and including lost time at work. The Committee is concerned only with quality of care. This is not a judicial or disciplinary process. Other factors surrounding the complaint are not within the Committee purview (thank goodness).

The examples I use are not extreme; they are typical. The common theme is that these are just citizens with the average dental IQ. The processes they complain about are often technically complex, difficult to undertake and hard to explain. The wonder is that there are not more misunderstandings.

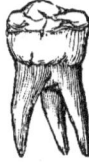

Foreword

I graduated from the University of Washington School of Dentistry in 1960 and spent the next forty years as a solo general practitioner, followed by five years with an associate who eventually bought my practice. During those forty five years I was fortunate enough to have a broad range of experiences, including:

- More than four decades as a member of a restorative dentistry study group, with a focus on crown and bridge.
- Five years as a clinical instructor at the UW Dental School in Restorative Dentistry.
- Member of the Board of Directors of the WSDA malpractice company, 1989-2000.
- Member of the Board of Trustees of the Washington Dental Service Foundation, 1992-2001.

- Along the way I was president of my local dental society as well as the State Association.

In the year 2000, I was hired by Washington Dental Service as the Associate Dental Director, a part time position which included various activities as a contact with the dental practice community. That position changed in 2009 and I took on some new responsibilities, including the examination and summarizing of complaints from patients about their dental care. It was an ideal fit, as far as I was concerned. It was a chance to utilize all those years of experience with multiple thousands of individuals and hundreds of thousands of procedures.

Relatively few of the situations described in the complaints I have reviewed are foreign to me. Additionally, I seem to recognize many of the complaining people, or at least their personality type. Dealing with complaints has provided me with a surfeit of amusement, nostalgia, annoyance, and a renewed sense of amazement at the ability of some individuals to rationalize their behavior and to attach the most base of intentions to the actions of others.

These years of reviewing the complaints made by patients about dentists has led me to a couple of conclusions:

    a. The whole world may not be filled with unhappy patients, but there is a significant number that are dissatisfied with the dental care they have received, and...

b. Sometimes they have good reason (but more often they are uninformed or confused or just pissed off).

A few reasons for all the unhappiness:

1. Dentists can be less than clear in explaining a particular treatment and all the post-operative possibilities.
2. Dental patients, like consumers everywhere, often hear what they want to hear and remember what they want to remember.
3. Unhappy patients always want (a) a refund, (b) someone other than the original dentist to repair/redo the treatment in question, and (c) someone (DDWA, the insurance commissioner, the Better Business Bureau, the FBI, the United Nations) to investigate the dental office and level punishment.
4. These disputes often take on the look and feel of an ugly divorce, with all sorts of side issues dragged into the complaint.
5. In the majority of the cases I have reviewed, the problem was bad communication and unrealistic expectations. However, sometimes the dentist has screwed up. It happens. We will look at some of those cases as well.

        – Curtis. F. Smith, DDS

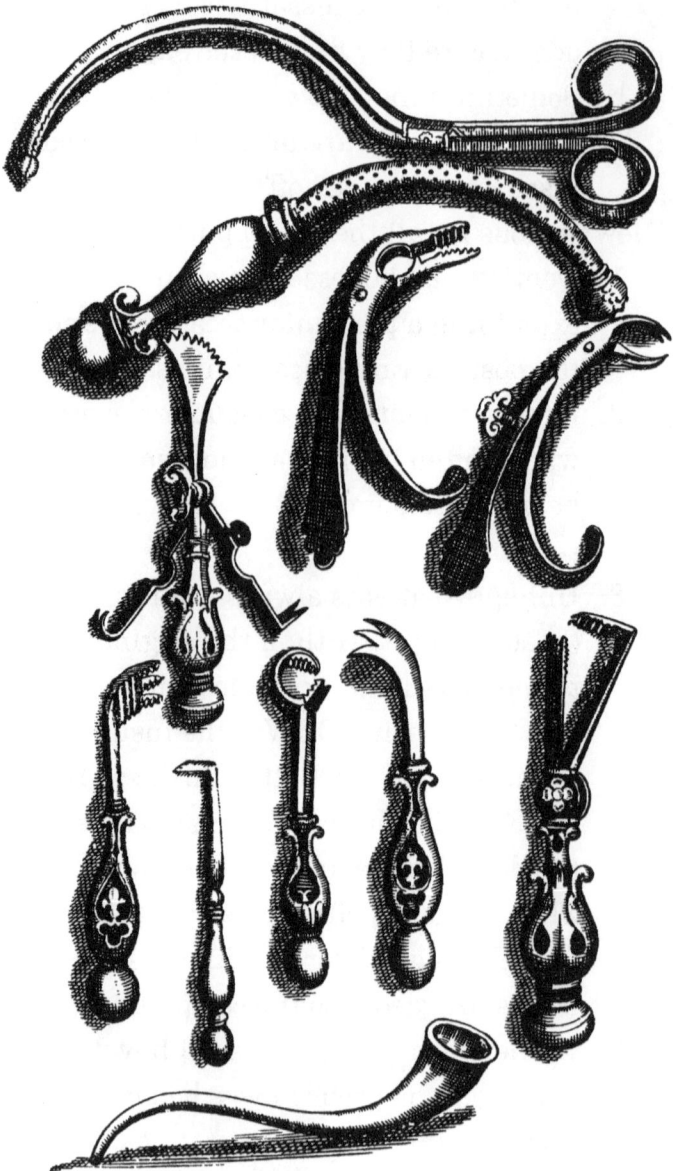

Dental surgery & related instruments from
"Armamentarium Chirurgicum," an important text of the time
by Johann Schutes (1595-1645) an Ulm physician.

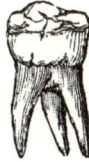

Chapter 1

Confusion

Confusion is certainly a common ingredient of many complaints. It becomes **the central issue** when it cannot be overcome with an explanation and applied logic.

Occasionally, a patient will latch on to an idea or opinion and become unshakable in their attachment to it. For instance:

Ms. M:

A fixed bridge on the upper right side became the subject of a deadlock. Ms. M refused to pay her portion of the fee for the restoration because "the teeth are too big." Of course, the size of the teeth in the three-tooth bridge is controlled by the width of the available space and the length necessary to meet the lower teeth. The size is really not negotiable, but it became the sticking point, with the patient refusing to pay for her portion of the fee after the insurance claim had paid. It was only resolved when she was convinced that there would not be another insurance benefit available for a second bridge.

And faulty memory can complicate things as well:

Roberta L:

Complaints can sometimes suggest that the patient resides in an alternative universe. In this case the problem is with a lower fixed bridge, which the patient says was placed by the dentist (Dr. L), 11 years ago. Dr. L graduated from dental school nine years ago, established his practice and Roberta became an early patient. There is no payment of a claim for the bridge in insurance company records and no entry in her dental chart for the bridge. It is unknown what dentist actually placed the bridge and when it was done.

Roberta's medical history suggests that treatment may face an array of hurdles. The medical complications include: lupus, osteoporosis, myocarditis, narcolepsy, mitral valve prolapse and acid reflux. The medication list is equally daunting.

Because she has an inexpensive HMO-type policy, the benefit available to replace the bridge is limited to the cost of a lower partial denture, which would be a considerable step down, functionally from a bridge and a hefty cost which would be born by Roberta. She remains convinced, all evidence to the contrary, that Dr. L placed the bridge and should therefore replace it at no cost. Thus is raised a point seen in many of the complaints stemming from unhappy patients. It goes something like this: "You worked on this tooth so you are now responsible for any further treatment needed, regardless of timing or cause."

Occasionally a simple misunderstanding can evolve in strange ways. This complaint illustrates just such an unexpected outcome.

Mr. S:

Mr. S. thought he needed four restorations, three at his first appointment, then one at the second. He made the co-pay payment for all four. When he arrived for the second appointment he was surprised to find that he had three more to do and owed co-pays for all of them.

The dental chart shows that four fillings were done at appointment one. Both treatment plans were signed by Ted.

After spending considerable time examining the chart and treatment plans, Ted declared that his signature had been forged. He went so far as to bring a police officer into the dental office to show him the alleged forgeries. The officer declined to become involved, stating that this was a civil matter. The QM committee noted that their purview does not extend to involvement in criminal matters. The complaint was tabled. What resolution was arrived at is unknown.

Ms. E:

This case demonstrates confusion on all the parties involved. Since only two teeth are named, it seems that the confusion potential is limited, but those involved are inventive.

The teeth that are the subjects of this complaint are the upper centrals, #8 and #9. The patient's mother, Ms. E, insists that the wrong tooth, #9, was crowned by Dr. B. She goes on to claim that the crown was seated incorrectly and as a result, has a cavity.

The dental chart and the claim record show that tooth #8 had a crown placed and tooth #9 received a composite restoration. This appears to be a mistake in the dental office record keeping, as there is a photo showing tooth #9 with a crown and #8 in need of composite fillings. Tooth #9 had been previously treated with a root canal, and it is likely the crown was placed because of aesthetic issues.

In 2017, Dr. J placed a crown on tooth #8. The

crown claim was denied because a claim had been paid only one year previously for a crown on that tooth.

Ms. E is now convinced that she has paid for three crowns and that one has a cavity. There have been only two claims for crowns. The claim confusion was sorted out and both crowns were paid. As to the concern about a cavity on one of the crowned teeth, no such problem was identified by either dentist.

Lest you think that confusion is always on the part of the patient, this story will disabuse you of that notion. This happens more than it should.

Ms. M:

A crown was billed for tooth #30 on Ms. M. The actual crown was placed on tooth #31, but not billed. Ms. M did not pay her portion of the bill for the crown. She then moved to Dr. B's office complaining of a fracture of tooth #30. A crown was placed, but there was no benefit because the history showed a crown on that tooth. Tooth #31 needed a root canal filling, which was done. The crown on the tooth was replaced. There was a benefit for both the RCF and the crown.

A requested refund for the replaced crown was denied because Ms. M did not pay her part of that fee. (The front office finally figured out what happened and corrected the record.)

If you followed all that you should probably consider applying for a job with a dental insurer.

Occasionally, what might be attributed to patient confusion can be explained as neurosis/psychosis or perhaps attempted fraud.

Ms. H:

The case required an extraordinary amount of time, tracing through six years of chart notes, plus information from several other dental offices. What emerged was a picture of a very demanding patient who rejected treatment recommendations, changed providers repeatedly and asked the dental office to fraudulently change treatment dates to accommodate her financially.

The issue is a crown placed by Dr. B on a lower molar. She insists that it is "too tight," causing pain and sensitivity. She has been advised by two dentists that it is impossible for a crown that fits onto a tooth to be "too tight," and that the tooth needs endodontic treatment. She rejects those opinions and continues her insistence about the crown which she wants to have remade at Dr. B's expense.

Now and then there is a cultural component to a complaint. Familiarity with other cultures is useful in those situations.

Mr. L:

Mr. L is from Peru. All of his previous dental care was done there and he still travels there on occasion.

The complaint involves a cantilevered bridge attached to tooth #4 and replacing #5. Tooth #4 has a root canal filling in place. When Mr. L saw Dr. D, the crown on #4 had come off. Dr. D explained that the design of the bridge was not the standard in the United States. He recommended that the bridge be remade with abutments at #4 and #6. Mr. L declined that treatment and asked to simply have the crown re-cemented. After removing some occlusal caries, Dr. D did as requested.

While Mr. L was back in Peru, tooth #4 fractured off at tissue level. He consulted several dentists there who were in agreement that it was Dr. D's fault. (They should know, since they have been at it so much longer than we have. The Inca were doing dental procedures over a thousand years ago.)

The complaint asks for: (1) an attorney, paid for by dental insurance, to sue for malpractice; (2) return of money charged to dental insurance; and (3) repair of all damage caused by Dr. D.

The request was denied by the QM Committee.

Dr. E:

The patient is an Eastern European physician. The dentist, Dr. D, has tried to deliver dental care according to American standards. Dr. E is insisting that the existing root canal fillings, which are obviously inadequate, do not need re-treatment. Also, that a retained primary root and an impacted permanent cuspid can be left; and that the cantilevered bridge which has fallen off need not be replaced with a more structurally sound design, but simply re-cemented. He is asking for a refund for charges so far, so that he can seek treatment elsewhere.

The existing charges are for examination, x-rays and a prophy. No refund was allowed. It will be interesting to see where his treatment is done. He may have to return to Bulgaria.

Ms. B:

This case is unusual in that it had already been seen by the Dental Quality Assurance Committee, a state agency (DQAC). Their finding was that no further action was necessary.

The complaint is that an inadequate sealant on the lingual of tooth #7 caused the tooth to become non-vital. There are two problems with this opinion: (1) Sealants are not done on anterior teeth. They are done on bicuspids and molars to seal the occlusal (chewing surface) grooves to forestall a carious lesion; and (2) A sealant could not cause a tooth to become non-vital. That would require caries.

This had been explained to the family, but was not accepted. They still wanted Dr. S to pay for the root canal filling on tooth #7. They say that Dr. D, the dentist they self-referred to, told them that the sealant caused the tooth to be devital. Dr. D denies that quote. His chart notes state that he found no evidence of trauma and no caries.

The QM Committee agreed with the DQAC. No refund was authorized.

Now and then a little mystery creeps in to the QM process. For instance:

Ms. B#2:

The complaint involved a partially completed root canal filling on a lower molar. The dentist named was Adam Bunker. He was supposedly an associate in Dr. S's office. He was not listed on their website and the address on the complaint was not for Dr. S's office. The only Dr. Adam Bunker web listing in the nation is for an office in Clovis, New Mexico.

The tooth had two of the three root canals filled. Dr. Bunker (or whoever did the procedure) then referred Ms. B to Dr. S for completion of the treatment. She is asking for a refund for the partial treatment. There was a benefit for the completion of treatment and all the canals appear to be well filled. The QM Committee ruled that a refund was not justified, which was fortunate because Dr. Bunker appears to be a phantom and the address on the complaint was not for a dental office.

Sometimes, fear can be as bad as anger in making treatment difficult or even impossible. For instance:

Ms. R:

This complicated case involves a very fearful patient, five dental offices and reams of records. There are two porcelain crowns in the complaint, both done by Dr. C. Specifically at issue is the tissue level on tooth #7, as well as the crown contour, and a problem with #12 which is not spelled out. The tissue level on #7 is one that occasionally is seen where the margin of a new crown is exposed due to retreat of the tissue after crown preparation.

There are two possible treatments. Either redo the prep and make a new crown or do a gingival graft. In this case, treatment is complicated by the patient's concern about possible infection of the gingival tissue. She relates that a cousin became disabled as a result of such an infection. Her concern was so inflated that explanations and assurances were not effective. In fact, it became obvious that she was not capable of effectively cleaning around the two teeth which were involved in this case, because of her fear of possible infection.

There were several referrals, as surgery was considered, and those dentists' plans were explained and not accepted. Eventually Dr. C refunded the cost of the crown on #7 and dismissed Ms. R from his practice. The QM Committee decided not to become involved as it seemed unlikely that they could resolve the problem.

It's not unusual for folks who are really upset to be ignorant of what is actually going on. And sometimes the dental office is mistaken in their analysis of what is going on.

Mr. O:

Dr. M was treating Mr. O because Dr. B, his regular dentist, was not available due to vacation. A Cerec crown was placed on #3 after a fracture and there was a restoration done at the same time on tooth #5. Post-op pain began immediately.

The Cerec crown was replaced at the patient's insistence. Antibiotics were prescribed and endodontic treatment was discussed.

Pain persisted and there was a referral to an endodontist. After endo treatment Mr. O insisted that the whole problem was due to the original crown being made improperly. He demanded a refund and Dr. M agreed, even though it was obvious that the problem was in infected pulp, not a faulty crown. An office mistake led to a refund for the restoration on #5 as well, even though it was not part of the complaint.

The complaint asks for compensation for lost time at work plus pain and suffering. The QM Committee excused themselves from the process, pointing out the information on the complaint form, which states that only quality of dental procedures are to be considered.

Ms. M:

The complaint involves a fixed bridge placed by Dr. H while she was employed by a corporate dental office. There were problems with the occlusion in the area for an extended time after the bridge was inserted.

Eventually, the dental office replaced the bridge at a much reduced fee. By that time, Dr. H was no longer working at the dental office.

Ms. M filed the complaint, hoping to recover all costs for the bridge and also asking for a letter stating that Dr. H deliberately constructed the bridge so as to cause the occlusion problems. The dental office declined to produce such a letter and Ms. M refused to pay her outstanding balance to the dental office. She was dismissed from the practice. The QM Committee took no action on the complaint.

Sometimes a simple typographical error can lead to patient confusion. With a reasonable person, it can be corrected. Unfortunately, not everyone is reasonable.

Mr. F:

This is another referral case, this time for oral surgery. Mr. F arrived at the surgeon's office with a referral slip stipulating extraction of tooth #11. Tooth #11 is the upper left cuspid or canine. Removal of cuspids can lead to an array of problems both aesthetic and functional and is avoided wherever possible. Fortunately, the surgeon checked back with the referring dentist, questioning whether the tooth number was correct. The typo was discovered and changed to #10.

Correcting Mr. F's opinion of which tooth was to be removed was not so simple. He steadfastly remained convinced that it should have been #11, and refused to be swayed by the explanations made by the two dental professionals. So, he filed a complaint. That didn't change the facts of the case, but presumably he felt better. Everybody was a winner. The dentists avoided a potentially problematic extraction, Mr. F got the treatment he needed and he got to complain about it.

Ms. P:

The treatment plan in this case was complex and involved a number of decisions regarding which teeth to retain and what treatment would be required for the various options. According to the dentist and the office manager, Ms. P initially seemed to understand the explanations made and the choices required.

As time passed she apparently became confused and/or forgot those discussions. Eventually she made the complaint. She stated that her initials on chart pages where treatment decisions were recorded were forgeries. One particular issue was her desire to not lose more teeth. When some were extracted, with her initials made on the chart page, she later insisted that she did not approve the extractions.

It would be hard enough if the only problem was the charge of forged initials. Here there was the added problem of a patient absolutely convinced that the treatment was not what she approved. A move to another dental office is the only answer. Based on the facts of this case, it seems likely that, in a few months, there will be another complaint from Ms. P.

Which tooth was treated by what dentist and when, often becomes the basis for a complaint. As noted in an earlier example, the tooth number can become part of the faulty memory. Another example:

Ms. K:

We start with a patient recollection that a crown was placed on tooth #12 in May 2011. There is no record in the claim history, nor in the dental charts of Dr. V, that a crown was placed on tooth #12 on that date. Tooth #12 was extracted in July, 2012 after a fracture made it unrestorable. There was a crown placed by Dr. V for Ms. K in 2011. It was on tooth #10. This was a devital tooth with a root canal in place. There was discussion of the small and short root, but Ms. K insisted and the crown was done, with a post and core in the root. That seems to be the tooth which has been confused with tooth #12.

Ms. K moved to the office of Dr. N, where an implant and crown were placed in August 2013 at the site of tooth #12. In April, 2014, Dr. N advised removal of tooth #10 because of increasing mobility. That led to a complaint from Ms. K, insisting that the crown had been placed on tooth #12 in May 2011. She was wrong about the tooth number and forgot the warnings about the ability of the root to support the crown.

Ms. W:

The complaint involved occlusal sealants placed by Dr. C in 2013. Two years later Dr. F again sealed those teeth. Ms. W is asking for a refund for the 2013 sealants, noting that they did not last.

I guess that every dentist has had to explain, probably more than once, that sealants are not permanent restorations. They can and will wear off. Their real purpose is to seal the grooves on the chewing surfaces of posterior teeth. I can be extraordinarily hard to determine whether those grooves are still sealed. To be safe, the sealant is usually redone. No refund was approved.

Treatment is often postponed if the patient is extremely apprehensive. That almost never makes things better and it did not in this case:

Ms. D:

A lower molar was causing discomfort, but Ms. D put off making an appointment until it was extremely painful. The decision was that tooth #18 needed a root canal filling. That was done by Dr. C, but, unsurprisingly, there was still pain in the area due to inflammation.

During instrumentation the end of a file broke off. Ms. D was told that it happened and it was possible to fill successfully around the file. Ms. D became convinced that the pain was because of the broken file. She requested a referral to an endodontist and saw Dr. T, who examined x-rays of the tooth and told her that the filling was fine and the file could not cause pain from inside the root. She was not satisfied with that assurance and contacted Dr. E, who retreated the root containing the file at her insistence. The pain gradually subsided, which it doubtless would have done irrespective of added treatment.

An interesting finding after all that is that no claim was received by the insurance company for any of the treatments to the tooth. Ms. D's request for a refund was moot. No payment, no refund.

Now and then there is a complaint that reflects more than average annoyance. The language can reflect just how upset the patient is. These folks are...

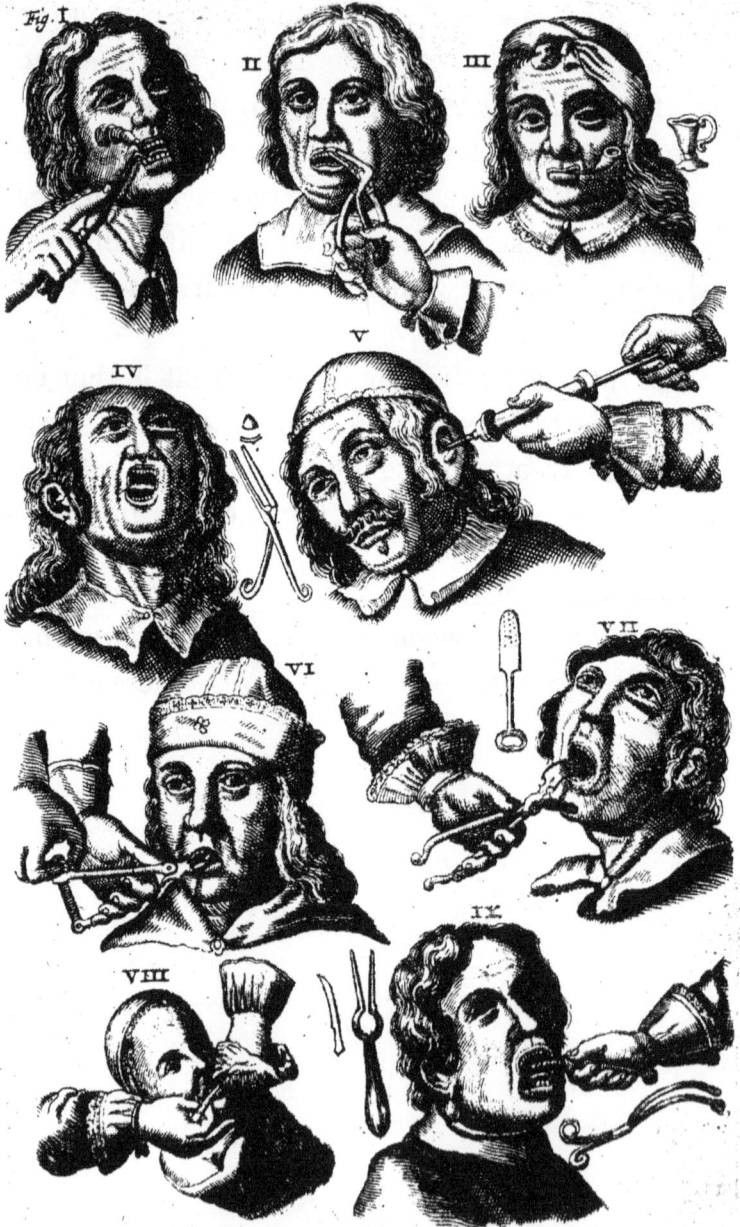

Dental & related operations from "Armamentarium Chirurgicum,"
an important text of the time by Johann Schutes (1595-1645) an Ulm physician.

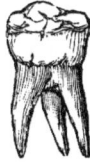

Chapter 2

Pissed!

Here are a few actual quotes:

"...they can expect me and a few others to protest in front of their building. They didn't tell me they were going to use dead man's bone in my mouth after pulling teeth."

(Note: dessicated human bone is sometimes used to help restore normal ridge contours after surgery.)

"... exposing the root lets in bacteria that could go to my heart. It's practically committing murder!"

"... so I would like a full refund for medical negligence that he put me through. Second of

all, I also had to get the work redone and I had to pay out of my pocket for that..."

(This was regarding a root canal filling that had to be retreated. The dentistry had been done in Mexico. The QM Committee has no authority in foreign countries.)

Ms. S:

The patient has complex dental issues. She refused Dr. G's recommendation of a upper full denture and lower partial. She wants no crowns. The eventual treatment plan was for upper and lower all acrylic partials, plus nine composite restorations. Shortly after the partials were inserted, she returned them, stating that she could not wear them. Another plan was offered which included a fixed bridge on the upper. She refused that plan as well.

A refund for monies received by the office from Care Credit required a form be signed. She refused to sign and left the office. An outstanding balance was eventually written off. The complaint asks for a refund for all expenses involved. The QM Committee decided that the written off balance approximated the patient portion of charges for restorations, so no refund as owed.

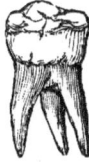

Chapter 3

And Sometimes, the Patient Is Just Wrong

Confusion can only explain so much. Sometimes patients manage to come up with ideas that are explained as normal post-op problems or are canceled by office records.

There is a tendency to forget or ignore the fact that procedures on humans are not always entirely predictable, as much as everyone involved would wish it were so.

Ms. R:

A root canal filling was done by Dr. A on a lower molar in 2009. There was a broken file left in one canal. The complaint states that Ms. R was not informed of the broken instrument. The tooth was retreated in 2012 by Dr. W. There was a benefit for that procedure.

The complaint is seeking $5000 from Dr. A for all charges from Dr. W including for the retreatment plus a payment for pain and suffering. Apparently, the note on the complaint form stating that claims for pain and suffering are not considered by the QM committee was ignored.

Broken instruments are recognized as a possible complication of root canal therapy. As long as the root can be sealed around the instrument fragment, it is not a problem. It is not possible for such a fragment, sealed inside a root, to cause symptoms. There is a chart note indicating that Ms. R was informed of the broken instrument. There is a signed form showing possible root canal complications. Broken instruments are listed.

The request for a refund was denied.

As mentioned earlier, patients sometimes hear what they want to hear. They can also come up with their own diagnosis:

Ms. S:

A crown was placed on tooth #31 in 2010. In 2017 the tooth became sensitive. The crown was removed to allow a root canal filling to be completed. There were delays in completing the root canal which amounted to five weeks. During that time the tooth was covered with a temporary crown.

When it was time to place the crown back on the tooth, it was determined that recurrent caries on a margin made a new crown necessary.

This allowed creative thinking to arise. The complaint was that "the root canal was not performed in a clean fashion" and therefore "my crown could not be used." Of course, caries does not become active in five weeks and certainly not when a temporary crown is in place, but what the heck. It's worth a try.

The S's:

Here we have Ms. S and her husband both complaining that the wrong tooth was treated with a root canal filling in spite of the x-ray evidence and the testimony of the referring dentist and the endodontist. When Ms. S insisted that the endodontist work on the tooth she thought was the problem, he pointed out that he had an obligation to work on the one designated by the referring dentist and that work had already started on that one. When last heard from, she was still convinced that she was right and the two dentists were wrong. She has moved on to another dental office. It might be interesting to find out how that is working out; then again, maybe not.

Ms. P:

Even though it was known that several anterior teeth needed treatment, Mrs. P. postponed appointments for several months until symptoms could not be ignored. Then, when treatment was started, she left the country on vacation for three weeks. Pain was ongoing during her vacation and until crowns were due to be seated, so root canal fillings were started for two teeth.

Having come up with the rationale that, since the root canals were just continued treatment, they should be done at no cost, she refused to acknowledge the charge for those treatments. Dr. M did not agree. At this point it is unknown how that worked out, but it was probably not amicable.

Ms. A:

The claim in this complaint is that coronal polishing by Dr. B's hygienist caused loss of the glaze on veneers of the upper centrals. The request is for Dr. B to pay for new veneers.

In reviewing the treatment history, it becomes clear that repeated suggestions that there should be a treatment plan established are dismissed by Ms. A. She also complains that her desire to discuss treatment are ignored. The chart notes show that she had two appointments to talk with Dr. B and failed to keep either one.

The date when the alleged damage to the

veneers supposedly occurred was Sept. 2007. The first chart note indicating she was not satisfied with the veneers was March of that year. At that time Dr. B informed her that the two incisors lacked adequate root length and were at risk of loss. He suggested replacement with implants, but again stated the need for a comprehensive treatment plan. There is then a series of six appointments when there is no mention of veneers in the record. The last appointment is February, 2008. She then moved on to another dental office.

The complaint was lodged in May, 2009, nearly two years after the alleged damage occurred. The QM Committee decided not get involved.

No refund.

Mr. H:

Mr. H is convinced, despite all evidence to the contrary, that a crown on an upper cuspid was not done by Dr. M in 2006. He is sure that it was done by a different dentist in 2001.

Dr. Miranda has supplied chart notes and a signed approval for the finished crown which prove it was done in 2006. Now, in 2012, it is time to replace the crown due to recurrent caries. There is a seven year replacement limit, meaning that Mr. H will be responsible for the cost without an insurance benefit. When it advantageous, memory can be selective.

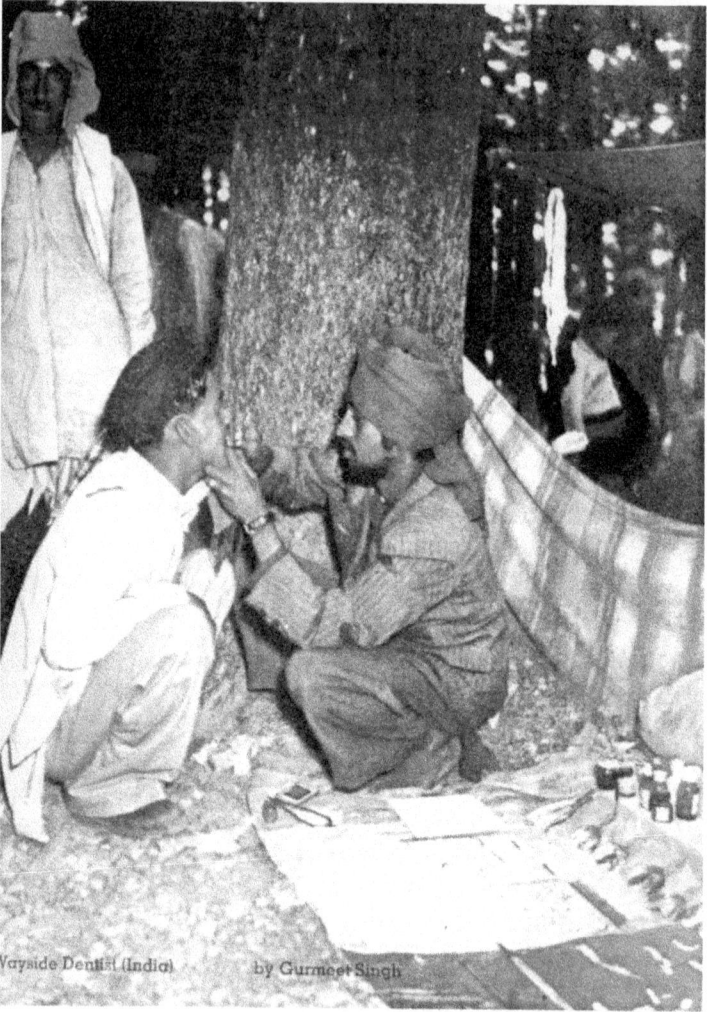

Vayside Dentist (India)   by Gurmeet Singh

Though modern methods reach primitive places, refinements are not yest available to all. This outdoor dentist's spread contains some medications, forceps for pulling teeth, impression trays for making models of teeth-lost jaws, and artificial teeth for dentures to restore them. Photo by Gurmeet Singh of wayside dentist (India) taken before 1969.

Ms. G:

This is a wide-ranging complaint touching on occlusion, post-op pain, extended anesthesia, a possible root canal filling and the fit of a retainer. A point-by-point denial from Dr. S proves that the claims are not only without merit, but apparently are not within the realm of possibility. His reply is as follows:

1. Extended anesthesia, cause unknown. Nerve damage would extend longer than 36 hours. This was an infiltration on the upper anterior. The anesthetic used has an average duration of 1-2 hours.
2. Post-op sensitivity is not unusual with composite restorations.
3. The composites on teeth #18 and 19 were on buccal surfaces. Interference with occlusion would have been impossible.
4. The ortho retainer in question does not contact the lingual surfaces of teeth #8 and 9. The labial wire does not contact the restorations.
5. Our office did not treat tooth #30. If a root canal is needed, it has no connection to our office.

It is not surprising, when a lay person becomes convinced that there is a problem with a technical procedure, to be mistaken about what the problem is. Trying to extend the criticism too far is a sure path to a complaint that is unbelievable.

Ms. M:

The complaint involves post-op pain from a tooth with a root canal filling done by Dr. P.

Ms. M became convinced that the problem was caused by cysts and not by her bruxing habit, which was pointed out as a possible problem by Dr. P and also by Dr. H, who placed a crown on the tooth. A night guard appliance to help with symptoms was suggested by both dentists and rejected by Ms. M.

After several years with no resolution of the pain from occlusion, Ms. M moved to the office of Dr. M. He referred her to an oral surgeon for extraction of the tooth. She reported after the extraction that "he found two cysts." A review of the surgeon's records did not reveal any reference to cysts discovered during the extraction. Conversations with the dentists involved did not find any reference to cysts. Where Ms. M's fixation on that pathology came from is unknown.

Mr. G:

A lower molar was restored by Dr. S in 2015 after removal of an existing silver alloy. A chart note states that "the restoration was quite deep and the pulp chamber was visible." Post-op pain was almost immediate and a root canal filling was done.

Mr. G was convinced that the tooth became devital as a result of an occlusal adjustment done by Dr. S in 2014. Dentists on the QM Committee agreed that it is not possible to cause pulp death when undertaking an occlusal adjustment. If it were possible, it would introduce an entirely new set of factors into diagnosis. Mr. G's opinion is just wrong.

Mr. B:

A lower molar crown was placed by Dr. K in 2007. Mr. B later moved from the area and became a patient in the Dr. L practice. In 2011 a carious lesion was found on the margin of the crown and it was remade. Mr. B told Dr. L that the crown was about eight years old. The claim was not paid, since the crown was only four years old. Mr. B filed a complaint, asking that Dr. K pay for the crown since the original was faulty.

The QM Committee decided that recurrent caries after four years cannot be blamed on Dr. K. No refund authorized.

Some cases are so far over the top, so far beyond what would be thought of as an average, reasonable, "make a refund and everybody is happy" complaint, that they belong in a special category. Every practitioner has met at least a few and they are always glad to see those folks in the review mirror. Among dentists they are:

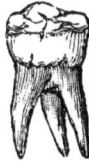

Chapter 4

The Patient From Hell (TPFH)

There is a common theme with the TPFH patients. Their complaints are long, detailed and emotional.

Ms. T:

Ms. T's complaint runs on for nine typewritten pages. It is a nearly day-by-day and hour-by-hour recitation of her symptoms and her interaction with the dental office. It is illogical, and at odds with the written record. There is, by several orders of magnitude, more information than is needed to describe problems with two full crowns. The crowns appeared to be clinically without any problems of fit or function. Ms. T is convinced the crowns are "too tight" and are causing the pain symptoms. It is impossible for crowns to be too tight. If they were too tight they would not seat fully on the tooth, which both of these crowns did.

Her tale is one of near constant pain involving both teeth. The chart notes show periods of no symptoms interspersed with a record of pain. Efforts were made by the dentist to address the pain symptoms when they occurred. When the problems persisted, she was referred to an endodontist (she failed to make an appointment there) and a TMD specialist (she made it to one appointment, then canceled on the advice of an osteopathic physician who doubted that mode of treatment).

Having received multiple post-op treatments at the dental office and essentially refused specialist treatment, Ms. T demanded a refund so that the crowns could be remade. There was no indication that a remake would address any problem, real or imagined, but the dental office did make a refund, just to be rid of her. The dentist who agrees to remake the crowns is either very brave or very foolish. The odds are that the whole miserable experience will be repeated.

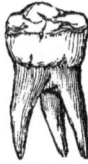

Chapter 5

The Uncooperative Patient

One of the phenomena most unexpected by me as a young graduate and neophyte practice owner was the occasional uncooperative patient. Foolishly, I assumed that Ms./Mr. and I were partners in dealing with whatever dental problem she/he presented. That was usually the case, *but* there were exceptions. It was one more instance that proved that in my late 20s/early 30s I still had a lot to learn about human nature. The good news is that it helped to prepare me for a lifetime of practice and years of dealing with complaints for a dental insurance company.

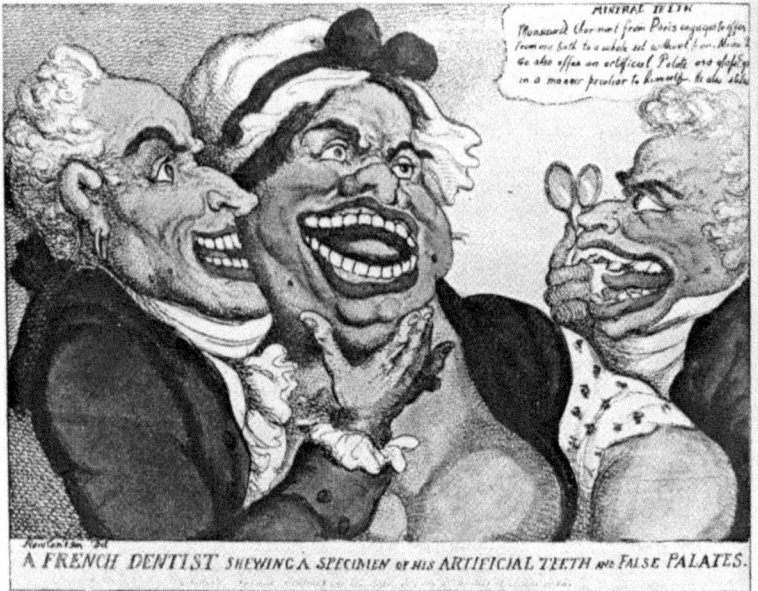

An engraving by Thomas Rowlandson (1756-1827), London, England.

When you combine misunderstandings and failed treatment with a lack of patient cooperation, the result is sure to be unfortunate.

Ms. C:

In this case there was preexisting periodontal disease which had been ignored for years. In addition there was a history of long-term tobacco use, carious lesions untreated, lost teeth resulting in no posterior occlusal support and generalized mobility of the remaining teeth.

Ms. C moved between two dental offices, apparently according to whim. The result was the lack of a consistent treatment plan. She refused to discontinue smoking and usually appeared only when in pain. This pattern continued for six years. At that point the complaint was filed.

There was no finding of below standard of care treatment.

Ms. B:

A complaint involving an immediate upper denture and a root canal filling plus crown, demonstrated just how uncooperative this patient could be. To be clear, an immediate denture (teeth are removed and the denture inserted the same day) is one of the most difficult procedures a dentist an take on. Combining that with a patient who does not follow instructions is not a path to success.

After receiving a schedule of post-insertion appointments, which are the period when the denture is adjusted and made comfortable, Ms. B did not return for ten months. At that time she was complaining of pain in a lower incisor.

Dr. K completed a root canal filling and placed a crown on the tooth. Ms. B refused a reline on the denture, but did sign a form indicating satisfaction with the crown. She again did not return for adjustments on the denture and a few months later filed a complaint asking for a refund for the denture and the crown. It seems that it would be impossible to be more uncooperative than that.

Ms. P:

Age can become an contributing issue if lack of cooperation is impacting treatment. In this case the patient is 86. She has had unsatisfactory interactions with several dentists in the community and has refused to pay for treatment rendered by at least two offices. She is now demanding replacement of an acrylic partial produced by Dr. E, with one that has a cast frame. Dr. E has offered to make a refund for the acrylic partial if it is returned, but since she has not paid him for it and it is in her mouth, it seems unlikely she will be tempted. There does not seem to be an obvious path to resolving this issue.

Lack of age can also be a problem when dealing with an uncooperative patient.

Ms. M:

This patient is now 19 years old. Her complaint (in part) reads, "Since I got my braces off when I was 15, my parents have not had time to take me to the dentist and I didn't always wear my retainer. Now my teeth have moved and Dr. B just says, 'you should wear your retainer.' Well yeah, but I need to get the teeth moved back, so I want to go to Dr. A to get it done. So please refund my money so I can get it done."

Young lady, I know this is an unwelcome move into the adult world, but you don't always get what you want if you have screwed up and not followed directions. Dr. B did his job, you didn't do yours. You don't get to have him pay to retreat your teeth. Welcome to adult responsibility.

Mr. W:

This complaint is remarkable primarily for its complete lack of connection to the actual facts as confirmed by chart notes and x-rays.

Mr. W contends that he requested treatment for a lower molar, but that Dr. P instead "extracted upper teeth because the compensation for those procedures was higher." There is a signed document requesting treatment for the upper teeth. There are other inconsistencies in the complaint which reveal that it is a work of fiction.

After repeated notices that payment for treatment would be expected when complete, Mr. W stated that he needed to go to a bank to withdraw funds. That was the last time that he was seen in the office.

The next contact was the complaint.

The request for a refund was not approved.

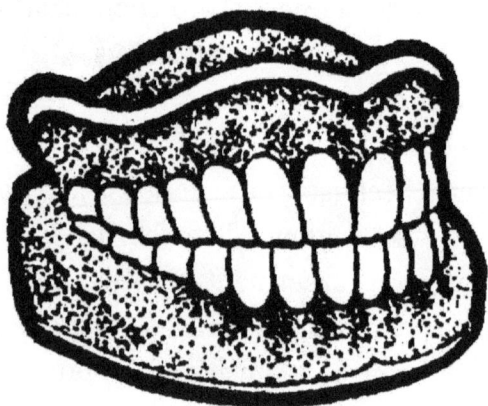

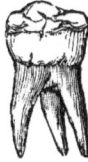

Chapter 6

Dentures: Immediate, Full and Partial

Replacing some or all of the teeth in an arch can be the most difficult challenge faced by a dentist. Some offices will simply not take it on, preferring to refer those patients needing dentures to a specialist. Issues with dentures account for more complaints than any other single category.

A few remarks about immediate dentures: The term "immediate" means that the teeth are extracted and the denture is inserted at one appointment. The difficulties are obvious. The denture is sitting on tissue that has just been the subject of trauma. The occlusion (the fit of the upper to the lower teeth) may be lacking. The denture can feel like a real mouthful. Everything hurts.

The reaction to this, which is often seen by the QM Committee, is the patient abandoning treatment at some point and moving to a different dental office because, "That guy didn't know what he was doing." The dentist may have known exactly what he was doing, but did not explain it well, did not prepare the patient for what was coming, or the patient just could not deal with the process. An immediate denture is not a pleasant procedure. It can often lead to a complaint.

Mr. J:

Occasionally, memory fails the patient and the question of what dentist made which appliance becomes muddled. In 2008, Dr. C made a lower immediate denture as a replacement for a lower partial. There was already an upper denture, made by an unknown dentist. Mr. J did not return for adjustments and treatment relines on the lower. In 2009, implants were placed on the lower arch, again by an unknown dentist.

Dr. C placed the attachments for the implants into the lower denture. Again, Mr. J did not return for adjustments of the lower.

In May, 2011, Mr. J had a different office construct new dentures, upper and lower. He asked for a refund from Dr. C for the existing dentures. Since Dr. C did not make the existing upper, that request was not considered. The lower denture was lost during the replacement process, making it impossible for the QM Committee determine what problem, if any, made a replacement necessary. The lower had served for three years, giving at least the appearance that it was satisfactory.

Ms. B:

In some cases the disappearance of a patient after dentures are inserted is a mystery, but not always. The chart notes in this case give a clue as to what is going on.

Immediate full dentures were inserted for Ms. B in January 2007. There was nothing else noted in the chart until May, when attempts were made to collect the past due balance on the account.

Dr. D sold the practice to Dr. S in early 2008. Ms. B reappeared in late 2008 and had Dr. S place soft liners in the dentures. When he was ready to place a hard reline in both in 2009, she complained that the dentures were really not satisfactory and wanted a new upper and lower produced. The complaint soon followed, asking for a refund for both.

It was decided that two years after the fact is too long a period for deciding whether dentures (that the patient has not paid her portion of the fee for) are satisfactory. No refund approved.

A difficult and/or demanding patient can make the process of denture production difficult. When input from a committee is added it can become impossible.

Ms. R:

The immediate denture proved not satisfactory for Ms. R. The fit, the finish, the setup all proved to be problematic. Dr. S started over with a new denture at no charge. At that point Ms. R recruited friends to testify as to the shortcomings of both dentures. Opinions were varied with no common theme. Everything was wrong.

After attempting to produce a denture setup that made everyone happy, Dr. S decided to cut his losses, refund the fee for the denture and send Ms. R (and her friends) on her way. It is unknown how this eventually turned out for Ms. R. One can only hope that she eventually abandoned the committee approach and found satisfaction with a perfect setup. The alternative would be eating without teeth, not a long-term solution.

The QM committee decided that there was no evidence that there was a problem with the standard of care. No refund was granted, which was the end of the issue for them.

Ms. J:

This complaint begins with the sentence, "The lower partial does not fit comfortably." This was surprising because the partial was entirely tooth supported, meaning that the partial behaves more like two fixed bridges than a typical partial denture which can move on one or both ends. A fixed attachment at four points limits the movement and makes the appliance much more stable. Sore spots are easily handled as well. There was a hint as to the real problem, however, with a comment in the response from Dr. H. He stated that Ms. J had complained about the lingual bar and the display of metal clasps on the abutment teeth.

Dr. H produced a substitute lower partial using a thin and broad lingual plate rather than the bulky bar and substituting non-metal clasps for the metal ones. Of course, that eliminated any profit from the treatment, but Dr. H decided it was better than having an unhappy patient.

Mr. Y:

The patient had prominent upper front teeth, called excessive overjet by dentists and "Bucky Beaver" by everyone else. The proposed solution; remove those teeth and insert a partial denture with a better tooth alignment. This was to be an immediate partial, with an eventual replacement when healing was complete.

Complaints began immediately. The saddle over the surgery site was uncomfortable, the lip had an awkward crease, the teeth were still too prominent, everything hurt. In spite of signed agreements describing the process and what to expect, Mr. Y became increasingly upset and eventually smashed the saddle with a hammer before moving on to the office of Dr. H.

After some time, a new partial was produced. Healing was far enough along to make the process much less painful. The teeth were in more or less ideal alignment and the lip looked as it should. Since a substitute partial was always part of the plan, there was a benefit paid and the three parties worked out the rest of the finances.

Ms. R:

An immediate denture was proposed by Dr. M and accepted by Ms. R. There was no realistic alternative, but there were problems anticipated, which were discussed in advance. The ridge was so low as to make retention of a denture problematic. Implants were discussed and rejected due to cost. When the denture was inserted the retention was less than ideal. After three months and several treatment relines, the problem was not resolved.

Once again, implants were suggested as a way to resolve the retention lack. The only alternative to that would be adhesive. Ms. R decided—in spite of a signed understanding that retention without implants would be problematic—that she wanted a refund because Dr. M's treatment failed. She wanted to go to another dental office for another try at a denture.

The QM Committee was not sympathetic. When a treatment is done, with appropriate warnings of possible problems and those problems make success elusive, a refund is not justified. It would be possible to make changes to the denture which would make a final result much more certain. Expense would be the patient's responsibility.

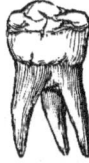

Chapter 7

Dental Care: Unlucky, Unfortunate, Unacceptable

Lest you think that all complaints are without merit, here are a few cases wherein the degree of technical skill and the soundness of judgment in planning treatment has been somehow questioned and the QM Working Group decided that a refund for treatment was justified.

This is a part of the patient's contract for dental care, which is there to guarantee that treatment is of recognized quality as determined by dental professionals' review. Fortunately, this kind of decision is reached in a minority of complaints and the number of complaints is a very small percentage of the total number of claims.

Ms. R:

Ms. R had a porcelain crown placed on tooth #2 by Dr. P. The crown broke, less than a year later. It was replaced at no cost. The replacement broke three years after it was placed. There was no benefit since a crown replacement is paid either after five or seven years, according to the contract.

This is an example of a recurring complaint, which is due to the preference for porcelain crowns by both dental offices and patients.

Broken porcelain crowns are among the majority of complaints received. The cost of gold alloys used to make full crowns has risen considerably in recent years. Dental offices, in order to hold laboratory costs in check, have embraced porcelain as a substitute. The downside was predictable.

There are now porcelain types which promise to be more durable. The downside of that is an increased cost for stronger porcelain. Whether metal will be more cost competitive given those increased costs will interesting to observe.

Ms. G:

Dr. G (no relation) placed a porcelain crown on tooth #2 in 2011. A few years later he retired. In 2015, the crown fractured. Ms. G's opinion is that the crown was of poor quality and she wants a refund.

Actually, the crown lasted four years, which is pretty good for a porcelain crown. It's also beyond the statute of limitations for the QM process, but there is another, simpler option available.

When dentists retire, their malpractice insurance becomes a "tail policy," which covers operations at the end of their working careers. That is the best option for coverage of the various problems which can arise after retirement. Contacting whatever dentist took over the practice or the estate should make it possible to find out what insurance company to contact.

Mr. M:

A fixed bridge from tooth #2 to #6 was placed by Dr. P in January 2011. Five months later Dr. P suddenly died.

A group of Dr. P's friend took over the practice and finished up a variety projects. They kept the practice functioning until it was sold.

In 2012, the bridge failed due to a fracture. This is another example of why malpractice tail policies exist. The policy paid for a fairly complex replacement bridge and everyone was happy.

Ms. K:

Dr. P placed a composite filling for Ms. K in 2015. In 2016 it was breaking down and was replaced by Dr. K (no relation). There was no insurance benefit due to the history. Dr. P had disappeared and was rumored to be practicing in another state under a different name. (I'm not making this up.) Fortunately, the decision was made to restore the benefit and pay Dr. K. Sometimes these things work out.

Ms. T:

A crown was placed in 2015 by Dr. E. At the time Ms. T was living in Tennessee. She then moved to Minnesota. The crown lost retention, fell off and was destroyed when she bit down on it. She contacted Dr. E and was told that if she returned to Tennessee he would replace the crown at no cost. That would involve a trip of 1100 miles.

There is a back story. This is actually crown #2. Crown #1 was broken after only a brief time and was replaced. The two crowns lasted a combined 14 months, which tells you a lot about porcelain crowns.

Not being willing to make a trip back to Tennessee, Ms. T requested a refund from Dr. E. That was granted by the QM committee. We can only hope that this replacement is a metal crown so that there is a chance of survival.

Sometimes that which should be obvious is somehow dismissed. In this case, a suggestion that the patient visit the ER instead of checking symptoms in the dental office had near a catastrophic financial result.

Mr. H:

There was pain on the lower left side after seating of a crown on tooth #18. A phone call to the dental office described the symptoms as difficult swallowing and swelling in the neck.

Post-op pain after seating a crown is among the most common of dental symptoms and so routine as to lead automatically to a diagnosis of infected pulp and a need for a root canal filling. Somehow that was overlooked.

The suggestion was that the patient visit an ER for possible treatment. After cycling through the ER, a brief hospital stay and a CAT Scan, Mr. H received a bill for $1500. Then he had to have a root canal filling.

Hospital ERs are poorly equipped to diagnose and treat dental problems. Diagnosis is outside their area of expertise. They fall back on the heavy artillery of testing which will almost certainly not be useful.

We close this section with the most outrageous case of over-billing that I can recall. Not surprisingly, it came from California.

Mr. S:

Mr. S states that he was in the dental chair in Dr. Z's office for one hour. Dr. Z maintains that it was three hours. Irrespective of which time frame is correct, there was an amazing amount of dentistry billed.

Mr. S says that he requested an exam, x-rays and a prophy. In addition to that the dental office added: a complete set of periapical x-rays and a panelipse (full mouth) film; a full-mouth scaling and root planning (which would usually take 2 to 4 hours); 18 composite restorations.

The total billing for this $17,375.50. The insurance company actually paid $1,460, before they were informed of the facts of the case. Refunds were requested.

How this eventually worked out is unknown. Plainly, the insurance billing was a work of fiction. That dental office should be required to carry a warning label.

Some Final Thoughts

I think some reassurance is in order. Despite being somewhat immersed in complaints and some questionable treatments for a few years, I can assure anyone concerned about their dental treatment that they are in good hands. The overwhelming majority of dentists display an absolute devotion to quality treatment of your dental problems. They do this not only because of their concern for you, but because that attitude is part of who they are.

Of course, there are a few scoundrels, but you can recognize them if you pay attention. An inordinate concern with how much money is to be earned is a warning sign.

If you don't understand the treatment proposed, ask questions. If you have the right dentist he will be as committed to successful treatment as you are. Trust your instincts, but find a dentist that you can trust.

I wish you well, few dental problems and contentment. Keep flossing!

Acknowledgments

Thanks are due to Dr. Larry Kuhl, Dr. Ron Inge during his time with the company, and to Dr. Kyle Dosch, for their leadership and technical input regarding the QM process. In addition, the dental consultant staff members (Mike, Scott, Abbie, Kieran and Salma) who were drafted now and then into the Committee, gave invaluable perspective. The whole thing could occasionally become overwhelming due to voume and complexity. The teamwork made it less so. Thank you all.

Other Books by the Author

The Brothels of Bellingham,
A Short History of Prostitution
in Bellingham, WA
©2004, Curtis F. Smith, D.D.S.
ISBN: 0-939576-13-9
published by The Whatcom County Historical Society

A History of Washington Dental Service
Published internally in 2004,
the 50th Anniversary of the company.

About the Author

Curtis F. Smith was born and raised Bellingham, Washington. He graduated from Bellingham High School in 1953 and the University of Washington School of dentistry in 1960. He is a past editor of the "Washington State Dental Association News," and for several years was a community columnist for the *Bellingham Herald*.

www.ingramcontent.com/pod-product-compliance
Lightning Source LLC
Chambersburg PA
CBHW022130280326
41933CB00007B/625